DIALYSIS AND HAVE

CHRONIC KIDNEY

TABLE OF CONTENTS

INTRODUCTION:

Living with chronic kidney disease and requiring dialysis can be challenging, but proper nutrition can help to manage symptoms and improve overall health. A diet that is tailored to the needs of individuals on dialysis can help to maintain a healthy weight, regulate electrolyte balance, and reduce the risk of complications. To help individuals with chronic kidney disease on dialysis maintain a healthy diet, we have compiled a collection of recipes that are specifically designed for people with these conditions. These recipes are easy to prepare, delicious, and provide a range of nutrients that are important for maintaining health while on dialysis

CREAMY CHICKEN AND MUSHROOM SOUP

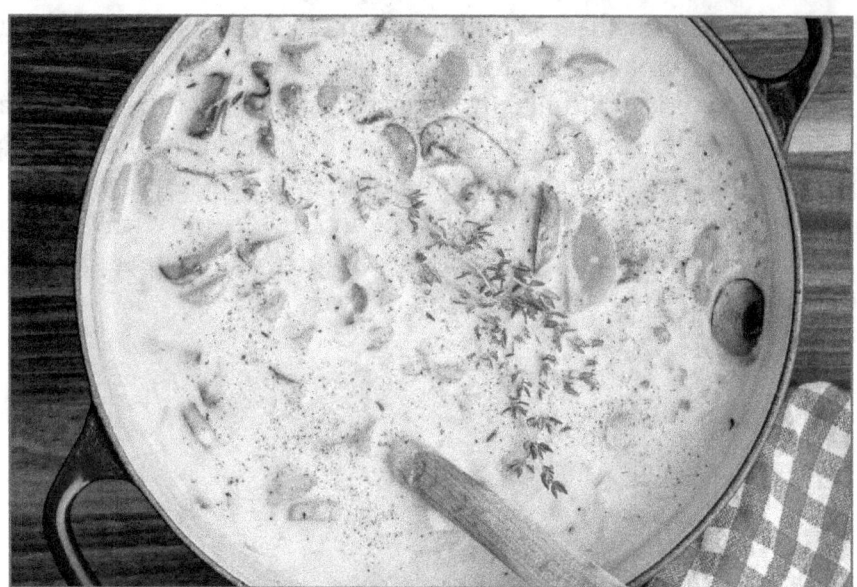

Ingredients:

- 2 tablespoons unsalted butter
- 1 onion, chopped
- 2 cloves garlic, minced
- 8 oz mushrooms, sliced
- 1 teaspoon dried thyme
- 4 cups low-sodium chicken broth
- 2 cups low-fat milk
- 1 lb cooked chicken breast, shredded
- Salt and pepper to taste

Instructions:

- ➢ In a large pot, melt butter over medium heat.
- ➢ Add onion and garlic, and cook until onion is translucent, about 5 minutes.
- ➢ Add mushrooms and thyme, and cook for another 5 minutes.
- ➢ Add chicken broth and milk, and bring to a simmer.
- ➢ Add chicken breast and cook until heated through, about 5 minutes.
- ➢ Season with salt and pepper to taste.

GRILLED LEMON PEPPER SALMON

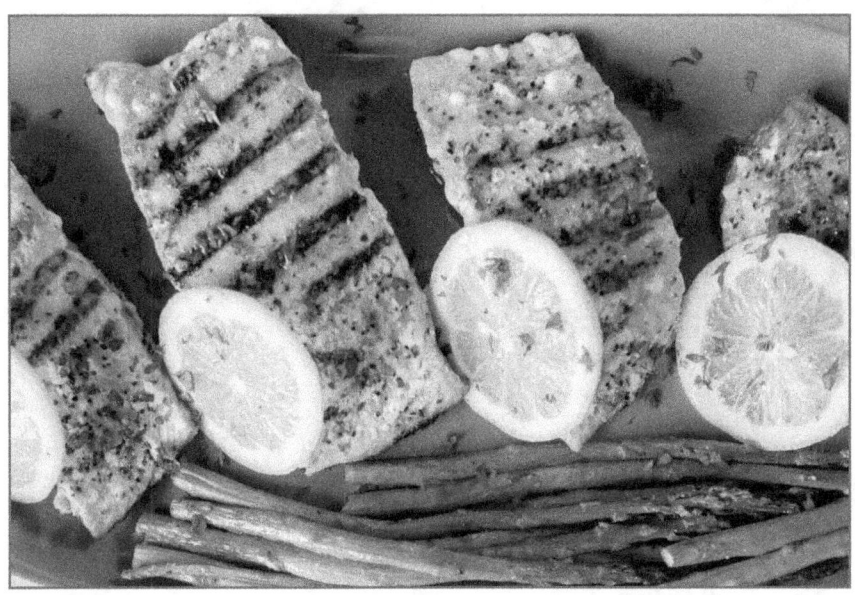

Ingredients:

- 4 4-oz salmon fillets
- 1 tablespoon olive oil
- 1 lemon, sliced
- 1 tablespoon black pepper
- Salt to taste

Instructions:

- ➤ Preheat grill to medium-high heat.
- ➤ Brush salmon fillets with olive oil.
- ➤ Season with black pepper and salt.
- ➤ Place lemon slices on top of salmon fillets.
- ➤ Grill salmon for 4-5 minutes per side, or until cooked through.

EGG WHITE OMELETE

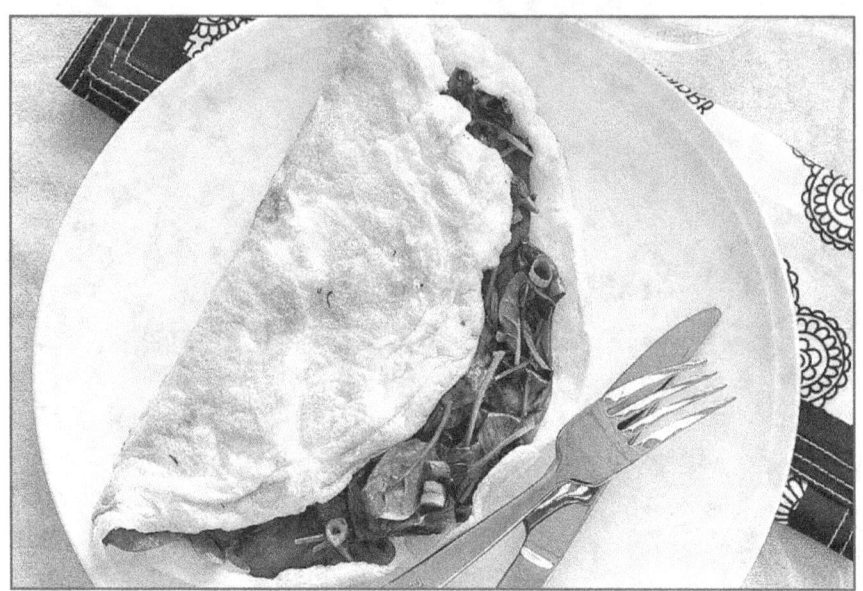

Ingredients:

- 4 egg whites
- 1 teaspoon olive oil
- 1/4 cup chopped spinach
- 1/4 cup chopped mushrooms
- 1/4 cup chopped bell peppers
- Salt and pepper to taste

Instructions:

- ➢ In a small bowl, whisk egg whites with salt and pepper.
- ➢ Heat olive oil in a non-stick pan over medium heat.
- ➢ Add spinach, mushrooms, and bell peppers, and sauté until vegetables are tender.
- ➢ Pour egg whites into the pan and let cook for 2-3 minutes, until the bottom is set.
- ➢ Fold the omelet in half and continue cooking for another 1-2 minutes.

QUINOA SALAD

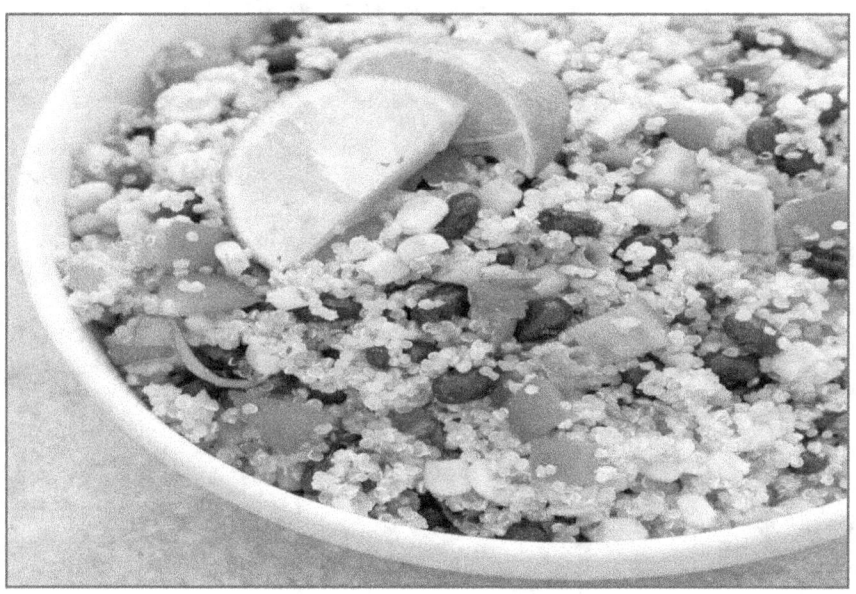

Ingredients:

- 1 cup quinoa, rinsed
- 2 cups water
- 1/2 cucumber, chopped
- 1/2 tomato, chopped
- 1/2 bell pepper, chopped
- 2 tablespoons chopped parsley
- 2 tablespoons chopped mint
- 1/4 cup olive oil
- 1/4 cup lemon juice
- Salt and pepper to taste

Instructions:

➤ In a medium pot, bring quinoa and water to a boil.
➤ Reduce heat to low, cover, and simmer for 15-20 minutes, until quinoa is tender and water is absorbed.
➤ In a large bowl, mix together cooked quinoa, cucumber, tomato, bell pepper, parsley, and mint.
➤ In a small bowl, whisk together olive oil, lemon juice, salt, and pepper.
➤ Pour dressing over quinoa salad and toss to combine.

BAKED CHICKEN AND VEGETABLES

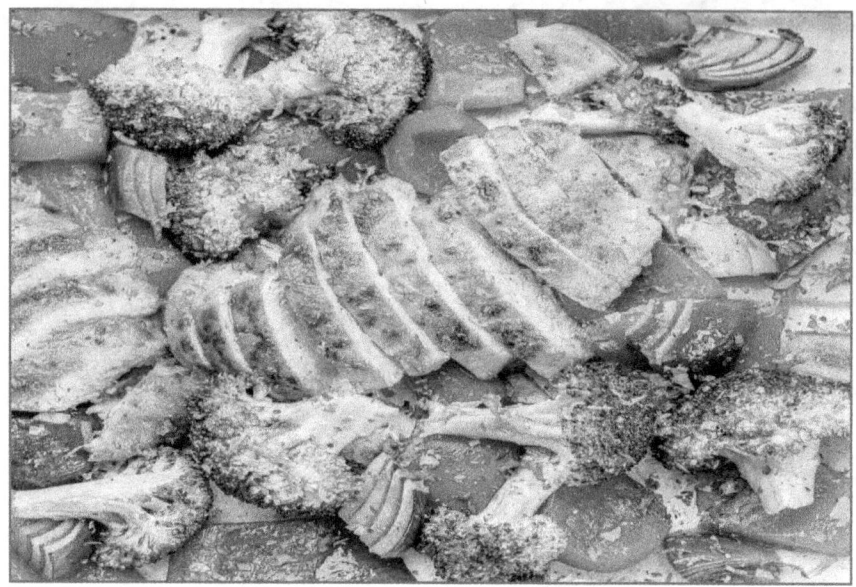

Ingredients:

- 4 boneless, skinless chicken breasts
- 2 teaspoons low-sodium seasoning
- 1 teaspoon olive oil
- 1/2 lb carrots, peeled and chopped
- 1/2 lb green beans, trimmed
- 1/2 onion, chopped
- Salt and pepper to taste

Instructions:

- ➢ Preheat oven to 400°F.
- ➢ Season chicken breasts with low-sodium seasoning and salt and pepper to taste.
- ➢ In a large bowl, toss carrots, green beans, and onion with olive oil, salt, and pepper.
- ➢ Arrange chicken breasts in a single layer in a baking dish.
- ➢ Surround the chicken with the seasoned vegetables.
- ➢ Bake for 20-25 minutes, until chicken is cooked through and vegetables are tender.

TUNA SALAD WITH GREEK YOGURT

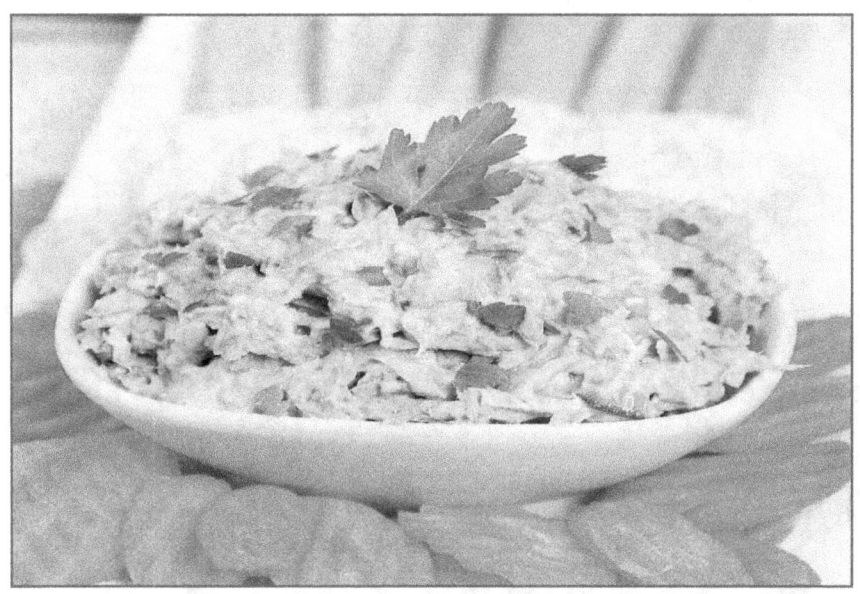

Ingredients:

- 2 cans of tuna, drained
- 1/2 cup plain Greek yogurt
- 1/4 cup diced celery
- 1/4 cup diced red onion
- 1 tablespoon chopped dill
- 1 tablespoon lemon juice
- Salt and pepper to taste

Instructions:

➢ In a medium bowl, mix together tuna, Greek yogurt, celery, red onion, dill, lemon juice, salt, and pepper.
➢ Serve over a bed of mixed greens or in a sandwich with whole wheat bread.

TURKEY CHILI

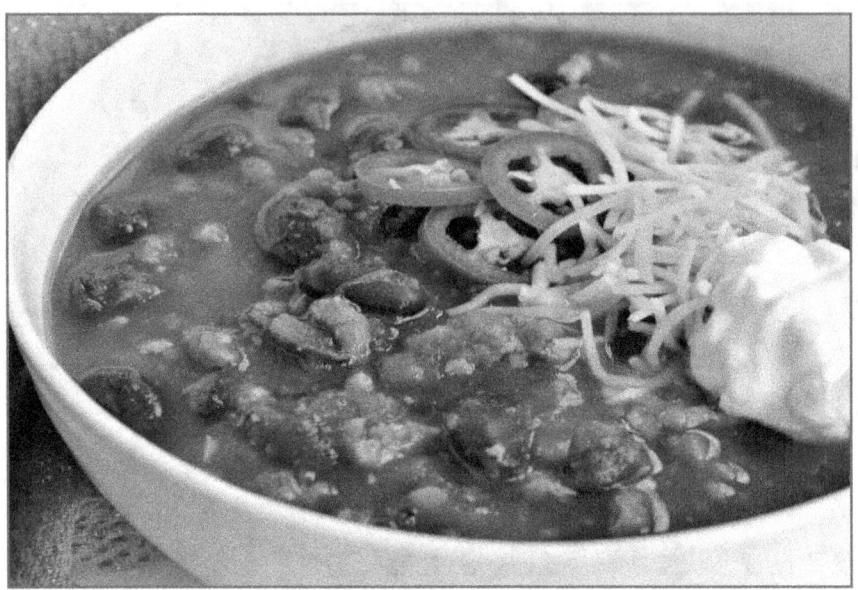

Ingredients:

- 1 lb ground turkey
- 1 onion, chopped
- 1 red bell pepper, chopped
- 2 garlic cloves, minced
- 1 tablespoon chili powder
- 1 teaspoon ground cumin
- 1/2 teaspoon smoked paprika
- 1/4 teaspoon cayenne pepper
- 2 cups low-sodium chicken broth
- 1 can kidney beans, drained and rinsed
- Salt and pepper to taste

Instructions:

- ➢ In a large pot, cook ground turkey over medium-high heat until browned.
- ➢ Add onion, bell pepper, and garlic, and cook for 5-7 minutes, until vegetables are tender.
- ➢ Add chili powder, cumin, paprika, and cayenne pepper, and cook for 1-2 minutes, until fragrant.
- ➢ Add chicken broth and kidney beans, and bring to a simmer.
- ➢ Reduce heat to low and let simmer for 15-20 minutes.
- ➢ Season with salt and pepper to taste.

LOW-SODIUM VEGETABLE SOUP

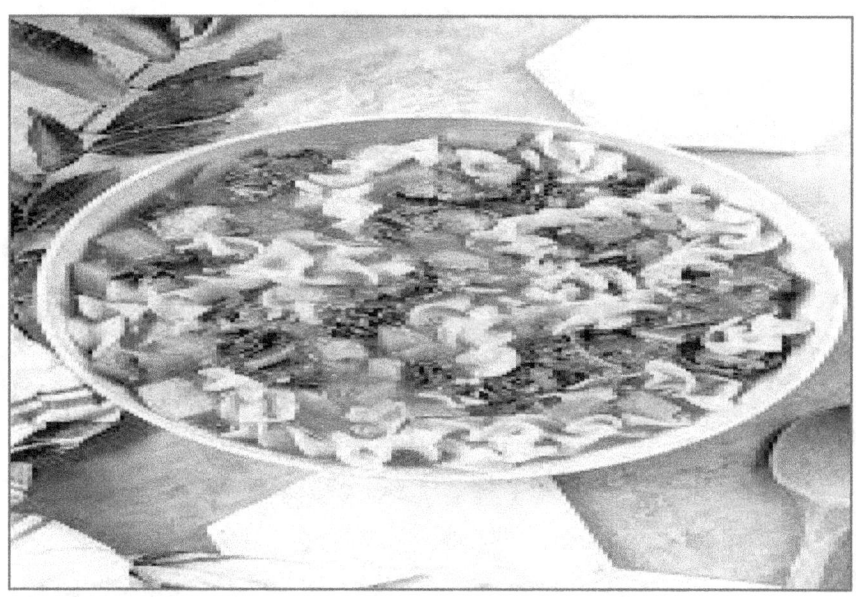

Ingredients:

- 2 tablespoons olive oil
- 1 onion, chopped
- 2 garlic cloves, minced
- 2 carrots, peeled and chopped
- 2 celery stalks, chopped
- 1 zucchini, chopped
- 1 yellow squash, chopped
- 4 cups low-sodium vegetable broth
- 1 can diced tomatoes
- 1 teaspoon dried thyme
- Salt and pepper to taste

Instructions:

- In a large pot, heat olive oil over medium heat.
- Add onion and garlic, and cook until onion is translucent, about 5 minutes.
- Add carrots, celery, zucchini, and yellow squash, and cook for another 5-7 minutes.
- Add vegetable broth, diced tomatoes, and thyme, and bring to a simmer.
- Reduce heat to low and let simmer for 15-20 minutes.
- Season with salt and pepper to taste.

ROASTED PORK TENDERLOIN WITH SWEET POTATOES

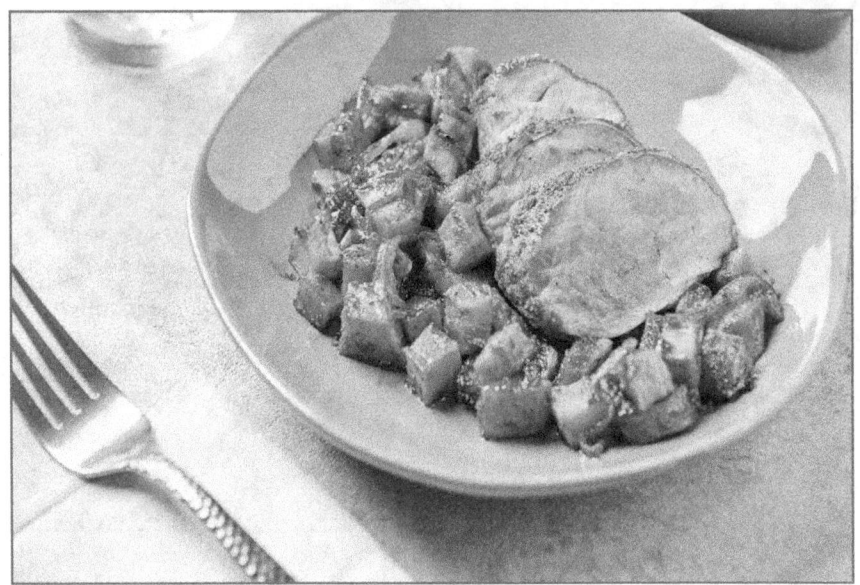

Ingredients:

- 1 lb pork tenderloin
- 2 sweet potatoes, peeled and chopped
- 1 onion, chopped
- 2 garlic cloves, minced
- 1 tablespoon olive oil
- 1 teaspoon dried rosemary
- Salt and pepper to taste

Instructions:

- Preheat oven to 375°F.
- In a large bowl, toss sweet potatoes, onion, and garlic with olive oil, rosemary, salt, and pepper.
- Arrange vegetables in a single layer in a baking dish.
- Season pork tenderloin with salt and pepper and place on top of the vegetables.
- Roast for 25-30 minutes, until pork is cooked through and vegetables are tender.

BAKED SALMON WITH LEMON AND DILL

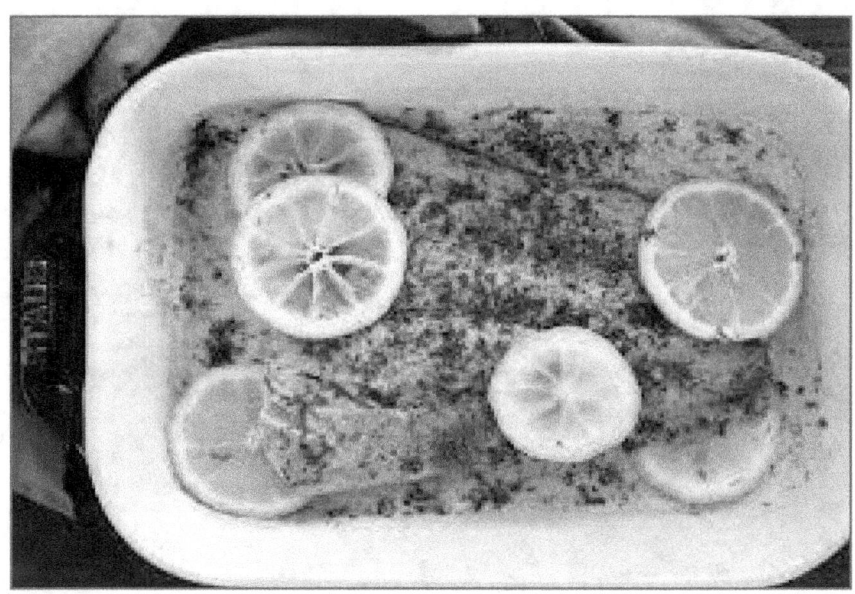

Ingredients:

- 4 salmon fillets
- 2 tablespoons olive oil
- 2 tablespoons lemon juice
- 2 tablespoons chopped fresh dill
- Salt and pepper to taste

Instructions:

- ➢ Preheat oven to 375°F.
- ➢ In a small bowl, whisk together olive oil, lemon juice, dill, salt, and pepper.
- ➢ Place salmon fillets on a baking sheet lined with parchment paper.
- ➢ Brush the lemon-dill mixture over the salmon.
- ➢ Bake for 12-15 minutes, until salmon is cooked through.

GRILLED SHRIMP SKEWERS WITH VEGETABLES

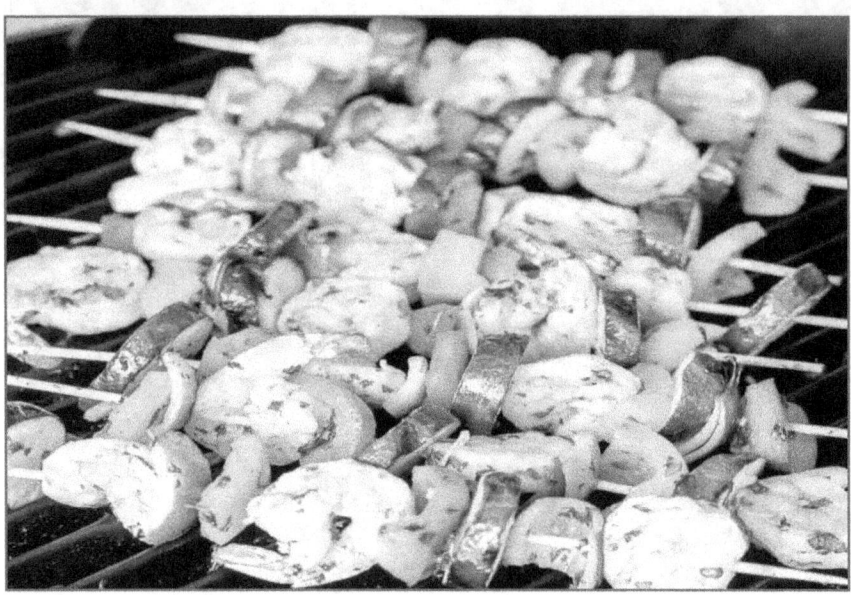

Ingredients:

- 1 lb large shrimp, peeled and deveined
- 1 red bell pepper, chopped
- 1 green bell pepper, chopped
- 1 zucchini, chopped
- 1 yellow squash, chopped
- 2 tablespoons olive oil
- 2 garlic cloves, minced
- Salt and pepper to taste

Instructions:

- ➤ Preheat grill to medium-high heat.
- ➤ In a large bowl, toss shrimp and vegetables with olive oil, garlic, salt, and pepper.
- ➤ Thread shrimp and vegetables onto skewers.
- ➤ Grill skewers for 2-3 minutes per side, until shrimp is pink and cooked through.

VEGETABLE AND CHICKEN STIR-FRY

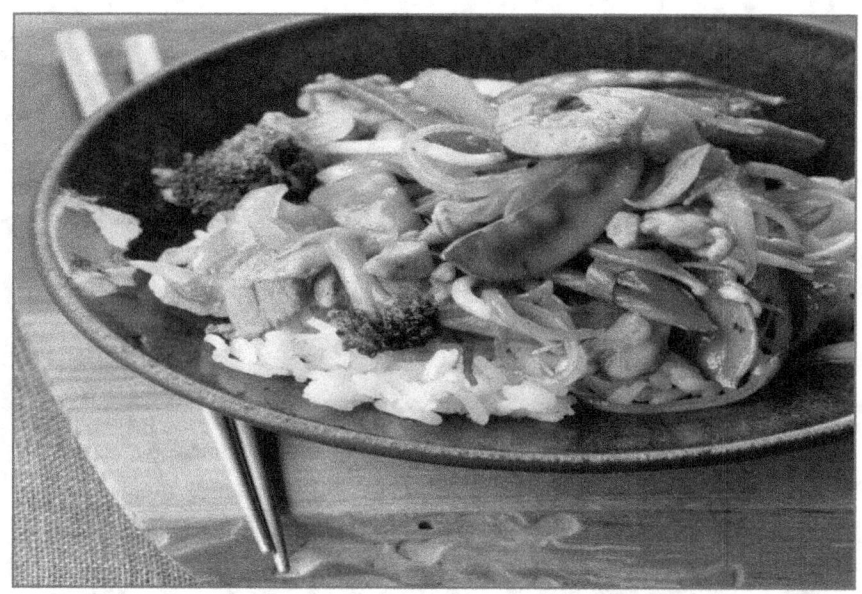

Ingredients:

- 1 lb boneless, skinless chicken breasts, sliced
- 1 onion, chopped
- 2 garlic cloves, minced
- 2 carrots, peeled and chopped
- 1 red bell pepper, chopped
- 1 green bell pepper, chopped
- 1 zucchini, chopped
- 2 tablespoons olive oil
- 2 tablespoons low-sodium soy sauce
- 1 tablespoon cornstarch
- Salt and pepper to taste

Instructions:

- ➤ In a large skillet or wok, heat olive oil over high heat.
- ➤ Add chicken and cook until browned on all sides, about 5 minutes.
- ➤ Add onion, garlic, carrots, and bell peppers, and cook for another 5-7 minutes.
- ➤ Add zucchini and cook for 2-3 minutes, until vegetables are tender.
- ➤ In a small bowl, whisk together soy sauce and cornstarch.
- ➤ Add soy sauce mixture to the skillet and stir until sauce thickens.
- ➤ Season with salt and pepper to taste.

QUINOA SALAD WITH ROASTED VEGETABLES

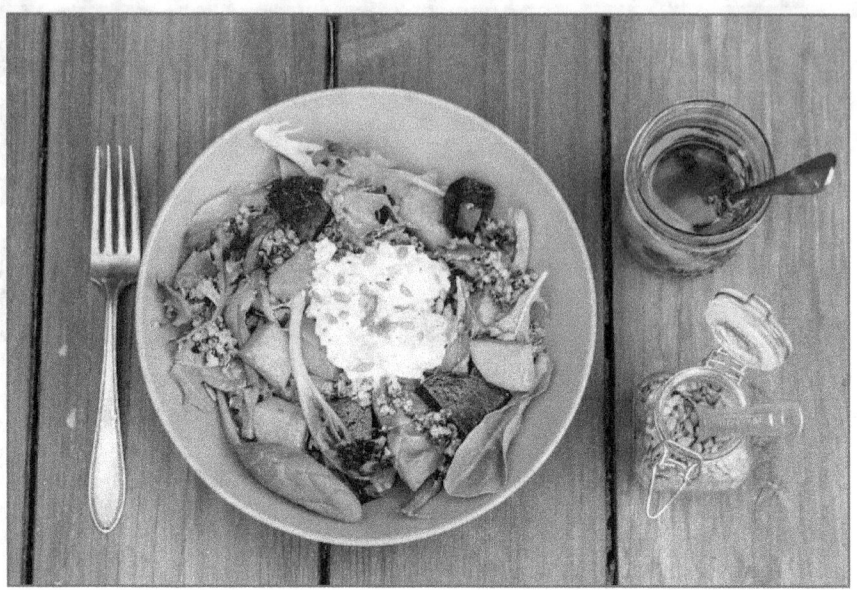

Ingredients:

- 1 cup quinoa
- 2 cups low-sodium vegetable broth
- 2 sweet potatoes, peeled and chopped
- 1 onion, chopped
- 1 red bell pepper, chopped
- 1 tablespoon olive oil
- Salt and pepper to taste

Instructions:

- ➢ Preheat oven to 375°F.
- ➢ In a large bowl, toss sweet potatoes, onion, and red bell pepper with olive oil, salt, and pepper.
- ➢ Arrange vegetables in a single layer on a baking sheet lined with parchment paper.
- ➢ Roast for 25-30 minutes, until vegetables are tender and lightly browned.
- ➢ In a medium pot, bring vegetable broth to a boil.
- ➢ Add quinoa and reduce heat to low.
- ➢ Cover and simmer for 15-20 minutes, until quinoa is cooked and liquid is absorbed.
- ➢ In a large bowl, combine quinoa and roasted vegetables.
- ➢ Season with additional salt and pepper to taste.

CHICKEN AND VEGETABLE SKEWERS

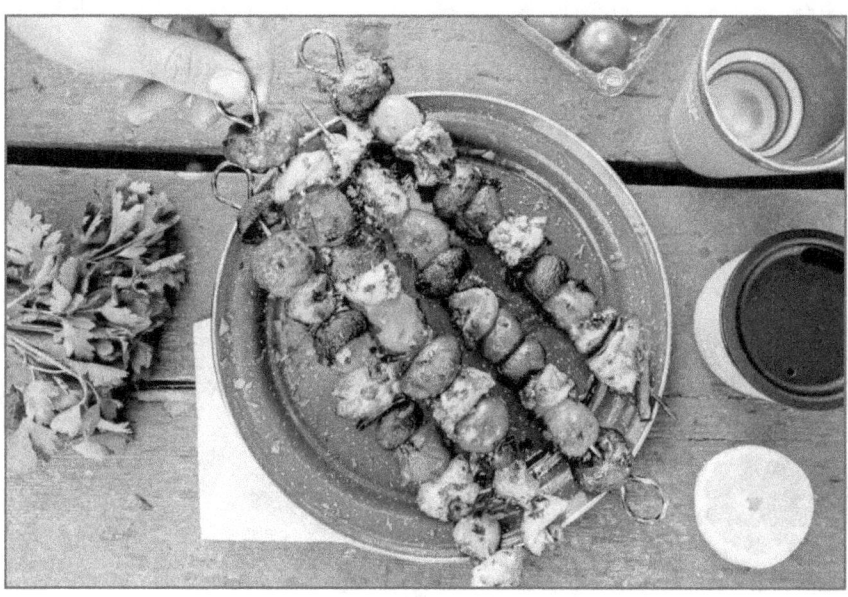

Ingredients:

- 1 lb boneless, skinless chicken breasts, cut into cubes
- 1 zucchini, cut into rounds
- 1 red onion
- 1 red bell pepper, cut into squares
- 1 yellow bell pepper, cut into squares
- 2 tablespoons olive oil
- 1 tablespoon low-sodium soy sauce
- 1 teaspoon garlic powder
- Salt and pepper to taste

Instructions:

- Preheat grill to medium-high heat.
- In a large bowl, whisk together olive oil, soy sauce, garlic powder, salt, and pepper.
- Add chicken and vegetables to the bowl and toss to coat evenly.
- Thread chicken and vegetables onto skewers.
- Grill skewers for 10-12 minutes, turning occasionally, until chicken is cooked through and vegetables are tender.

MEDITERRANEAN GRILLED CHICKEN

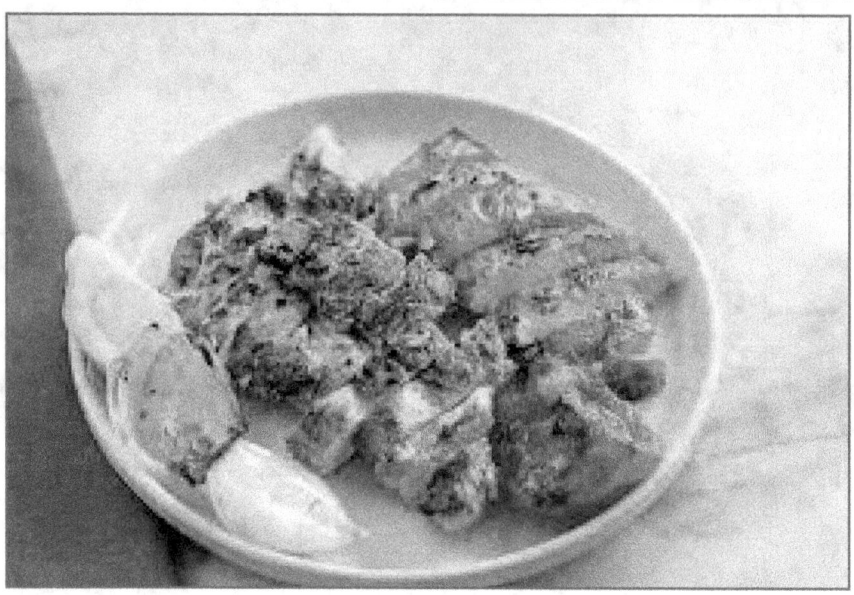

Ingredients:

- 4 boneless, skinless chicken breasts
- 2 tablespoons olive oil
- 2 garlic cloves, minced
- 2 teaspoons dried oregano
- 1 teaspoon dried basil
- 1/2 teaspoon dried thyme
- Salt and pepper to taste

Instructions:

- ➢ Preheat grill to medium-high heat.
- ➢ In a small bowl, whisk together olive oil, garlic, oregano, basil, thyme, salt, and pepper.
- ➢ Brush the mixture over both sides of the chicken breasts.
- ➢ Grill chicken for 6-7 minutes per side, until chicken is cooked through.

LEMON GARLIC SHRIMP

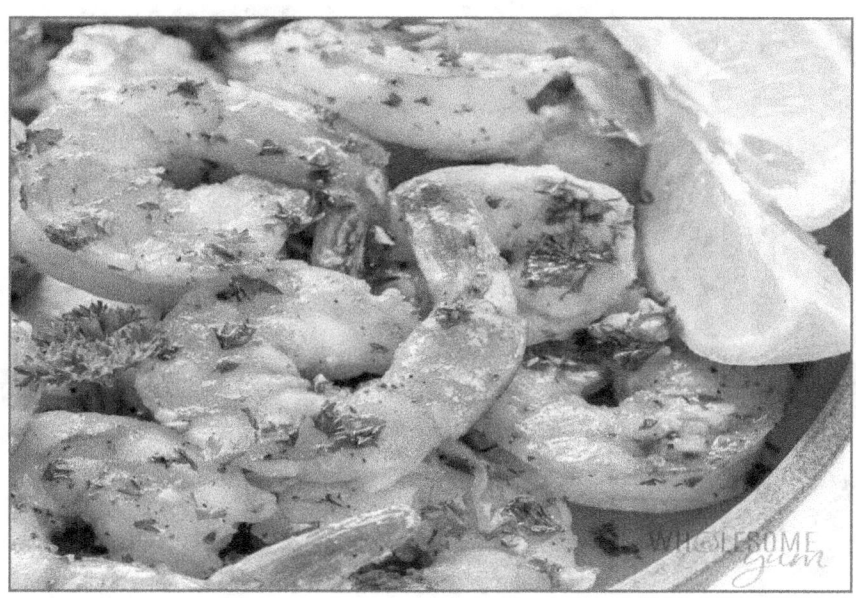

Ingredients:

- 1 lb large shrimp, peeled and deveined
- 2 tablespoons olive oil
- 2 garlic cloves, minced
- 1 lemon, juiced
- 1 tablespoon chopped fresh parsley
- Salt and pepper to taste

Instructions:

- ➢ In a large skillet, heat olive oil over medium-high heat.
- ➢ Add garlic and cook for 1-2 minutes, until fragrant.
- ➢ Add shrimp and cook for 2-3 minutes per side, until pink and cooked through.
- ➢ Add lemon juice and parsley to the skillet and stir to combine.
- ➢ Season with salt and pepper to taste.

TOMATO BASIL CHICKEN

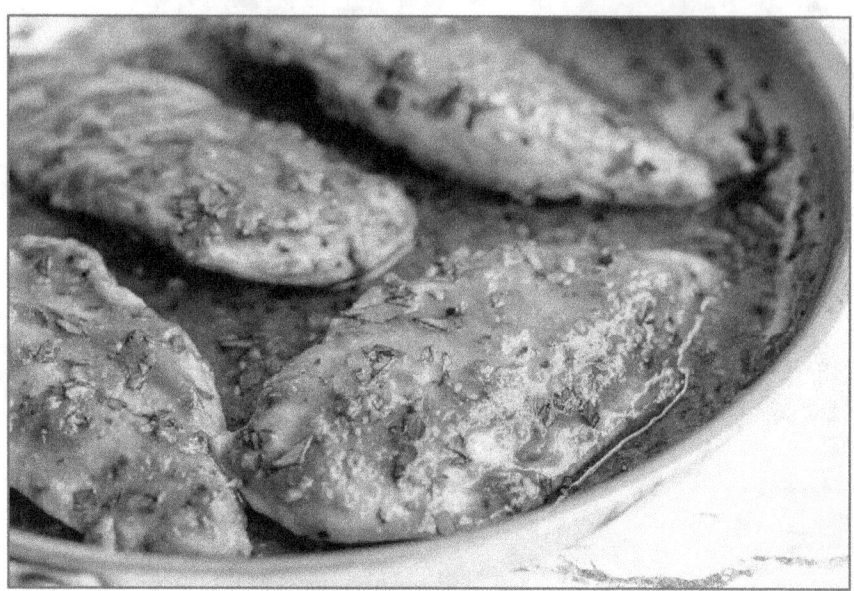

Ingredients:

- 4 boneless, skinless chicken breasts
- 1 tablespoon olive oil
- 2 garlic cloves, minced
- 2 cups cherry tomatoes, halved
- 1/4 cup chopped fresh basil
- Salt and pepper to taste

Instructions:

➢ Preheat oven to 375°F.
➢ In a large oven-safe skillet, heat olive oil over medium-high heat.
➢ Add garlic and cook for 1-2 minutes, until fragrant.
➢ Add chicken and cook for 3-4 minutes per side, until browned.
➢ Remove chicken from skillet and set aside.
➢ Add cherry tomatoes to the skillet and cook for 2-3 minutes, until they start to soften.
➢ Return chicken to the skillet and spoon tomato mixture over the top.
➢ Bake for 15-20 minutes, until chicken is cooked through.
➢ Sprinkle with chopped basil before serving.

LEMON HERB BAKED COD

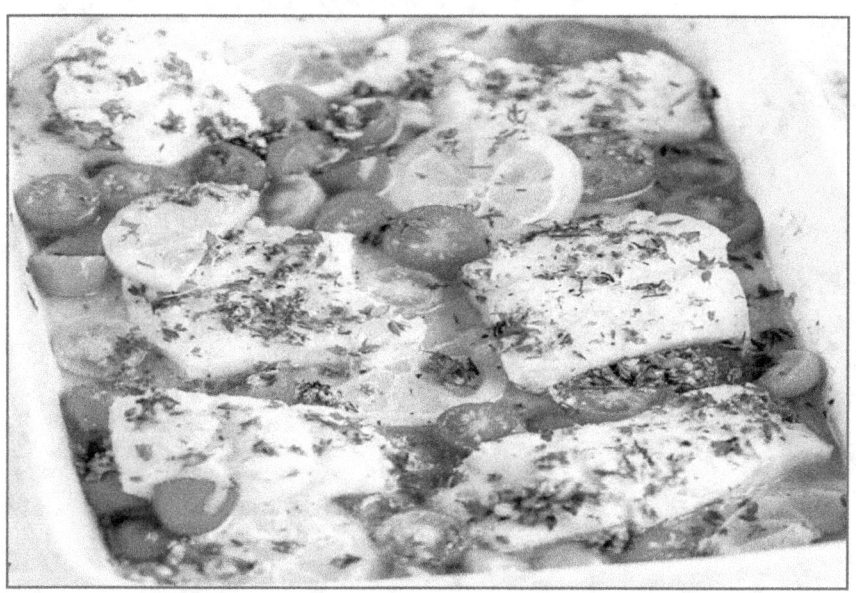

Ingredients:

- 4 cod fillets
- 2 tablespoons olive oil
- 1 lemon, juiced
- 2 garlic cloves, minced
- 1 teaspoon dried thyme
- Salt and pepper to taste

Instructions:

➢ Preheat oven to 375°F.
➢ In a small bowl, whisk together olive oil, lemon juice, garlic, thyme, salt, and pepper.
➢ Place cod fillets on a baking sheet lined with parchment paper.
➢ Brush the lemon-herb mixture over the top of the cod.
➢ Bake for 12-15 minutes, until cod is cooked through.

TURKEY AND VEGETABLE CHILI

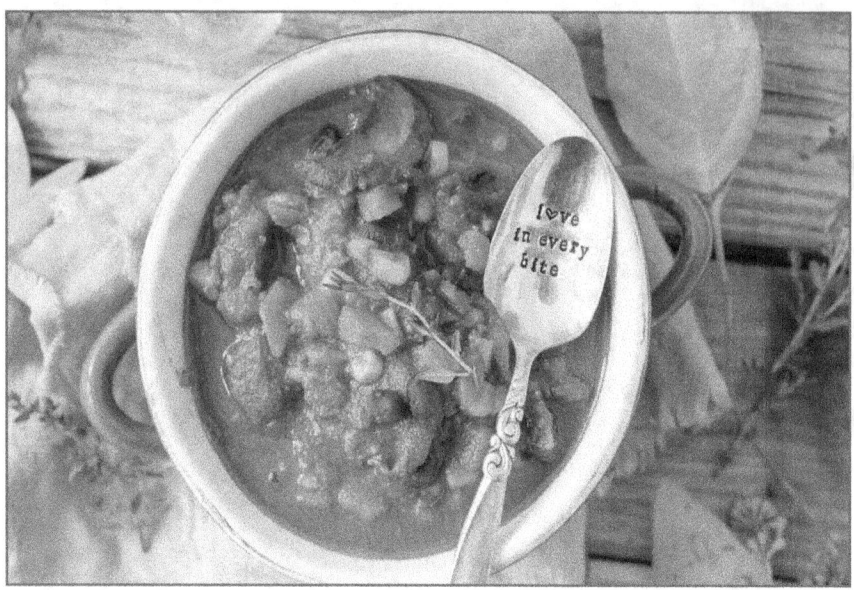

Ingredients:

- 1 lb ground turkey
- 1 tablespoon olive oil
- 1 onion, chopped
- 2 garlic cloves, minced
- 1 green bell pepper, chopped
- 1 red bell pepper, chopped
- 2 zucchinis, chopped
- 1 can (15 oz) low-sodium kidney beans, drained and rinsed
- 1 can (14.5 oz) diced tomatoes, undrained
- 1 cup low-sodium chicken broth
- 2 tablespoons chili powder
- 1 teaspoon ground cumin
- Salt and pepper to taste

Instructions:

- ➤ In a large pot or Dutch oven, heat olive oil over medium-high heat.
- ➤ Add onion and garlic and cook for 1-2 minutes, until fragrant.
- ➤ Add ground turkey and cook for 5-7 minutes, until browned.
- ➤ Add green and red bell peppers, zucchinis, kidney beans, diced tomatoes, chicken broth, chili powder, cumin, salt, and pepper.
- ➤ Stir to combine and bring to a boil.
- ➤ Reduce heat to low and let simmer for 20-25 minutes, until vegetables are tender and chili has thickened.

VEGETABLE STIR-FRY

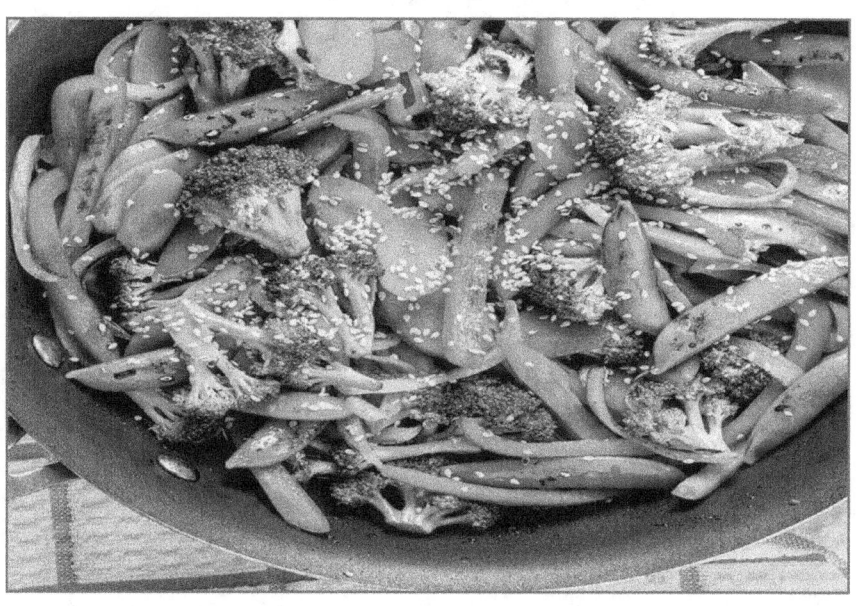

Ingredients:

- 1 tablespoon olive oil
- 1 onion, chopped
- 2 garlic cloves, minced
- 2 cups mixed vegetables (such as broccoli, carrots, snow peas, and bell peppers), chopped
- 1 tablespoon low-sodium soy sauce
- Salt and pepper to taste

Instructions:

- ➢ In a large skillet, heat olive oil over medium-high heat.
- ➢ Add onion and garlic and cook for 1-2 minutes, until fragrant.
- ➢ Add mixed vegetables and cook for 5-7 minutes, until vegetables are tender.
- ➢ Stir in low-sodium soy sauce and season with salt and pepper to taste.
- ➢ Serve over cooked brown rice or quinoa, if desired.

CONCLUSION:

A healthy diet is an essential component of managing chronic kidney disease and dialysis. By following these tips and trying out the recipes in our collection, you can enjoy delicious, nutritious meals that support your health while on dialysis. Remember to monitor your sodium intake, choose high-quality protein, be mindful of potassium and phosphorus, stay hydrated, and work with a registered dietitian to develop a personalized meal plan